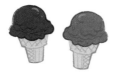

One Question a Day Journal for Kids

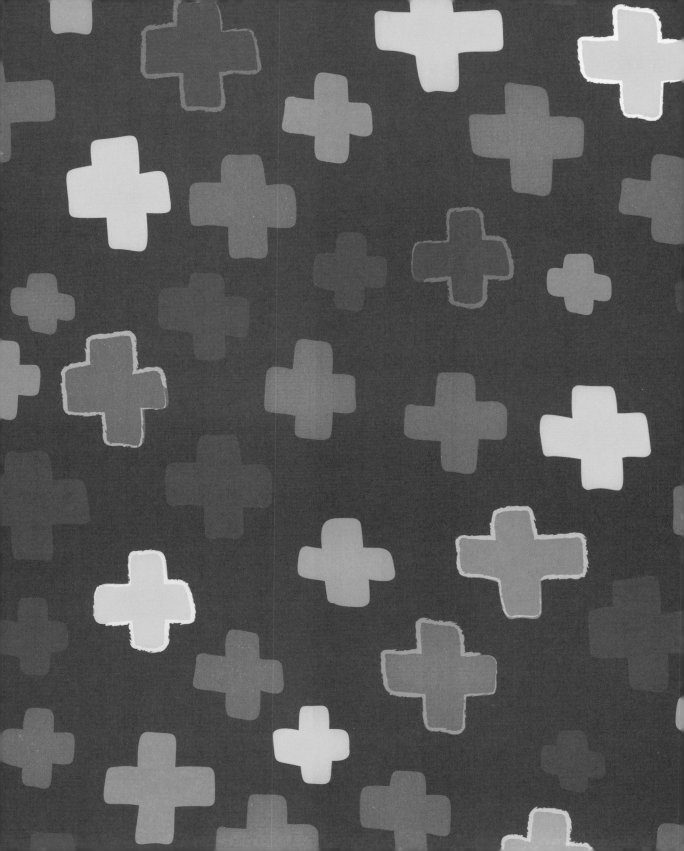

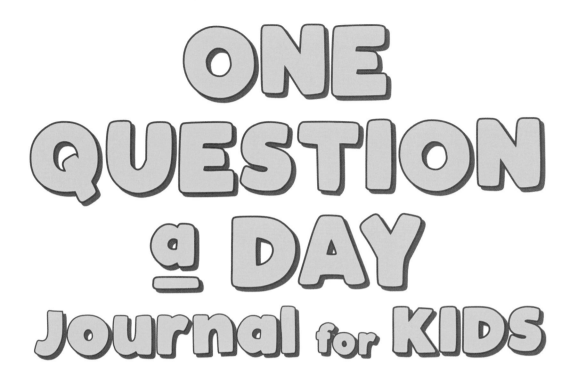

ONE QUESTION a DAY Journal for KIDS

365 Days All about Me

MaryAnne Kochenderfer, PhD

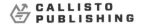
CALLISTO PUBLISHING

To Eva and Rachel,
and their brilliantly inquisitive minds

Published by Callisto Publishing LLC C/O Sourcebooks LLC
P.O. Box 4410, Naperville, Illinois 60567-4410
(630) 961-3900
callistopublishing.com

This product conforms to all applicable CPSC and CPSIA standards.

Source of Production: 1010 Printing Asia Limited, Kwun Tong, Hong Kong, China
Date of Production: March 2024
Run Number: 5038821

Printed and bound in China.
1010 22

This Journal Belongs to

. . . .

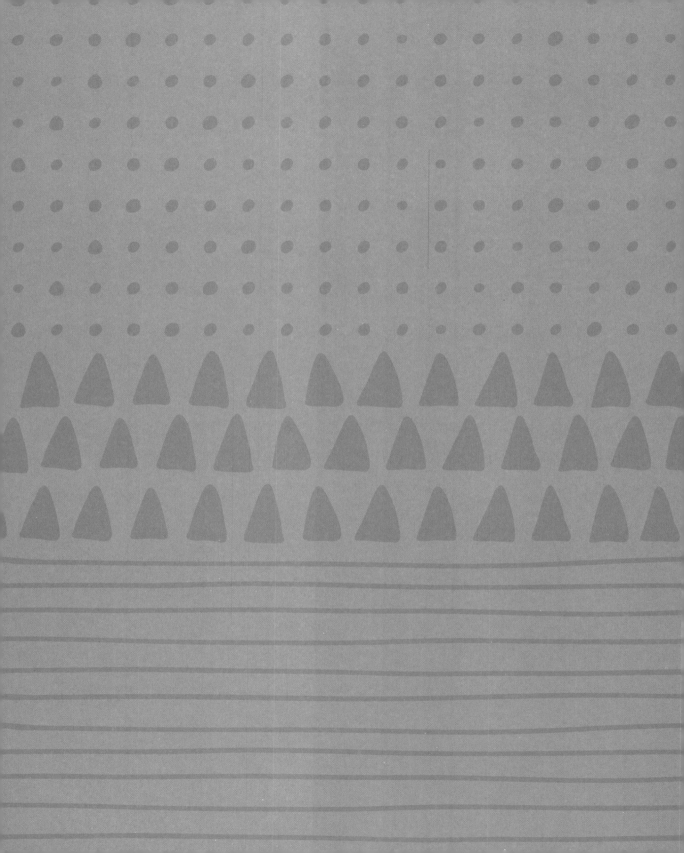

Introduction

Welcome to your One Question a Day Journal for Kids!

In this book, you'll explore all the amazing things about your life, including your favorite activities, the people you care about most, and lots of fun pretend topics that will get you thinking.

This book is designed to capture a piece of who you are right now and to create memories you can celebrate for the rest of your life! On these pages you'll find one question a day for 366 days. That's a full leap year! Or a regular year with a bonus question.

Writing in this book should be fun! Give your journal a special spot in your room and decide on a time of day when you'll write in it. Maybe you'll write first thing in the morning, right when you wake up. Or right before you fall asleep at night. Writing after dinner works, too—choose a time that works best for you. It's okay if you skip a day or if you're too busy to write an answer sometimes—you can always come back to it later. That's the beauty of keeping a journal—you can write however or whenever you'd like!

I hope you enjoy answering these questions and exploring the many things that make you so awesome. Don't forget to flip through this journal when you're done filling it out—you'll have so many amazing memories to remember.

Happy writing!

Day 1

DATE _____ / _____ / _____

What makes you happy and why?

_____

_____

_____

Day 2

DATE _____ / _____ / _____

What is your favorite activity when you have free time? What do you like about it?

_____

_____

_____

Day 3

DATE _____ / _____ / _____

Do you have a favorite song? How does it make you feel?

_____

_____

_____

Day 4

DATE _____ / _____ / _____

What do you look forward to the most every day?

_____

_____

_____

Day 5

DATE _____ / _____ / _____

Would you prefer to have long hair or short hair? Why?

_____

_____

_____

Day 6

DATE _____ / _____ / _____

What activities do you enjoy when it's hot outside?

_____

_____

_____

Day 7

DATE _____ / _____ / _____

What activities do you enjoy when it's cold outside?

_____

_____

_____

Day 8

DATE _____ / _____ / _____

What is your favorite animal? What do you like about that animal?

_____

_____

_____

Day 9

DATE _____ / _____ / _____

What would you like to invent someday and why?

_____

_____

_____

Day 10

DATE _____ / _____ / _____

What would your toys say if they could talk?

_____

_____

_____

Day 11

DATE _____ / _____ / _____

Would you keep a dinosaur as a pet? Why or why not?

_____

_____

_____

Day 12

DATE _____ / _____ / _____

How do you like to celebrate special occasions?

_____

_____

_____

Day 13

DATE _____ / _____ / _____

How old are you right now? What do you like about being this age?

_____

_____

_____

Day 14

DATE _____ / _____ / _____

If you had the ability to talk to and understand one kind of animal, which animal would you want it to be and why?

_____

_____

_____

Day 15

DATE _____ / _____ / _____

If you could be a character in a book or a movie, who would you be?

_____

_____

_____

Day 16

If you had a magic hat, what would its magical powers be?

_____

_____

_____

Day 17

How would your life be different if you lived underwater like a mermaid or a merman?

_____

_____

_____

Day 18

What is one thing that you do well?

_____

_____

_____

Day 19

DATE _____ / _____ / _____

If there was a secret passage near your home, where would you want it to lead?

_____

_____

_____

Day 20

DATE _____ / _____ / _____

Would you rather have a pet dragon or a pet unicorn? Why?

_____

_____

_____

Day 21

DATE _____ / _____ / _____

What do you like about your face?

_____

_____

_____

Day 22

DATE _____ / _____ / _____

If you were a butterfly, what colors would be on your wings?

_____

_____

_____

Day 23

DATE _____ / _____ / _____

What has someone said to you that made you feel happy?

_____

_____

_____

Day 24

DATE _____ / _____ / _____

Imagine you are as small as an ant. What would the world look like to you?

_____

_____

_____

Day 25

DATE _____ / _____ / _____

Who do you look up to? How would you like to be like them?

_____

_____

_____

Day 26

DATE _____ / _____ / _____

Would you rather live in a castle on a mountain or in a crystal palace underwater? Why?

_____

_____

_____

Day 27

DATE _____ / _____ / _____

If you could go back in time for one day, which period in history—and in which part of the world—would you visit?

_____

_____

_____

Day 28

DATE _____ / _____ / _____

If someone offered to sell you a piece of land on the moon, would you buy it? Why or why not?

.

_____

_____

_____

Day 29

DATE _____ / _____ / _____

If you were inventing an imaginary world, what is one way it would be different from our world?

_____

_____

_____

Day 30

DATE _____ / _____ / _____

Would you rather paint a picture or carve a sculpture? Why?

_____

_____

_____

"If you look the right way,
you can see that
the whole world is a garden."

—FRANCES HODGSON BURNETT, *THE SECRET GARDEN*

It's so exciting to see your thoughts on paper—keep it up!

Day 31

DATE _____ / _____ / _____

What do you like best about the place you live?

_____

_____

_____

Day 32

DATE _____ / _____ / _____

Who is your favorite famous person? What do you like about them?

_____

_____

_____

Day 33

DATE _____ / _____ / _____

If you were a wizard, what would your wand look like?

_____

_____

_____

Day 34

Think of a time when you did something nice for someone. How did that make you feel?

_____

_____

_____

Day 35

If you were asked to create a sculpture or a statue for the middle of your town, what would it look like? Why?

_____

_____

_____

Day 36

Would you rather write a book or film a movie? Why?

_____

_____

_____

Day 37

If you were a superhero, what special power would you have? What would you do with your power?

_____

_____

_____

Day 38

DATE _____ / _____ / _____

If you had a pet sloth, what would you name it? Why would you choose that name?

_____

_____

_____

Day 39

DATE _____ / _____ / _____

If you could give any gift to someone you care about, what would you give and who would you give it to?

_____

_____

_____

Day 40

DATE _____ / _____ / _____

Would you rather be able to fly or turn invisible? Why?

_____

_____

_____

Day 41

DATE _____ / _____ / _____

What is your favorite number? Why do you like that number?

_____

_____

_____

Day 42

DATE _____ / _____ / _____

What kind of job do you want when you grow up? Why?

_____

_____

_____

Day 43

DATE _____ / _____ / _____

What helps you feel better when you are upset?

_____

_____

_____

Day 44

DATE _____ / _____ / _____

If you could be the best in the world at something, what would it be?

_____

_____

_____

Day 45

DATE _____ / _____ / _____

If you found a mysterious, magical egg, what do you think might hatch from it?

_____

_____

_____

Day 46

If you were as tall as a giraffe, what would you see?

_____

_____

_____

Day 47

Is there something that someone you know can do that you would like to learn?

_____

_____

_____

Day 48

Imagine you are a squirrel. What kind of tree would you like to live in?

_____

_____

_____

Day 49

If you could magically solve someone else's problem, what problem would you solve?

_____

_____

_____

Day 50

If you could move to another country for one year, where would you go?

_____

_____

_____

Day 51

If you were an animal, would you rather be an animal that lives in a group or an animal that mostly lives alone? Why?

_____

_____

_____

Day 52

DATE _____ / _____ / _____

Would you rather be able to run really fast or draw really well? Why?

_____

_____

_____

Day 53

DATE _____ / _____ / _____

If you were moving to the planet Mars with your family, what would you take with you?

_____

_____

_____

Day 54

DATE _____ / _____ / _____

What is one of your favorite memories?

_____

_____

_____

Day 55

DATE _____ / _____ / _____

If you lived in a floating castle, what would you see beneath you?

_____

_____

_____

Day 56

DATE _____ / _____ / _____

If you planted a magic seed, what would grow from it?

_____

_____

_____

Day 57

DATE _____ / _____ / _____

What is your favorite way to show someone you love them?

_____

_____

_____

Day 58

How would you describe the place where you live?

_____

_____

_____

Day 59

Would you rather drive a race car or sail a sailboat? Why?

_____

_____

_____

Day 60

If you could try out three different jobs, what would they be?

_____

_____

_____

"At the end of the day, if I can say I had fun, it was a good day."

—SIMONE BILES

Great writing! This shows dedication.

Day 61

If you could share a magical object with one friend, what would you want the object to be?

_____

_____

_____

Day 62

What is a place you like to visit? What do you like about it?

_____

_____

_____

Day 63

If you could ride a unicorn, where would it take you? Why?

_____

_____

_____

Day 64

What is something you did to help someone recently? How did it make you feel?

_____

_____

_____

Day 65

Would you rather have an elephant or a monkey for a pet? What would you do with your new pet?

_____

_____

_____

Day 66

Would you rather ride a horse or fly an airplane? Why?

_____

_____

_____

Day 67

DATE _____ / _____ / _____

What is your favorite thing to do on a rainy day?

_____

_____

_____

Day 68

DATE _____ / _____ / _____

What do you think your life will look like when you are grown up?

_____

_____

_____

Day 69

DATE _____ / _____ / _____

What do you like about your school? If you could change one thing about it, what would you change?

_____

_____

_____

Day 70

DATE _____ / _____ / _____

How do you feel when you work hard on a project and are able to finish it? Why?

_____

_____

_____

Day 71

DATE _____ / _____ / _____

If you could ask anyone in history a question, who would you ask and what would you ask them? Why?

_____

_____

_____

Day 72

DATE _____ / _____ / _____

If you had magic shoes that could take you anywhere in the world in three steps, what is the first place you would visit? Why?

_____

_____

_____

Day 73

If you were an athlete, what sport would you play? Why?

_____

_____

_____

Day 74

If you could paint pictures on the walls of your room, what would you paint? Why?

_____

_____

_____

Day 75

What is something that happened this week that you would like to remember?

_____

_____

_____

Day 76

What does your favorite pair of shoes look like?

_____

_____

_____

Day 77

What are three colors that you like to wear? What do you like about them?

_____

_____

_____

Day 78

If you were a famous chef, what would be your favorite dish to cook? Why?

_____

_____

_____

Day 79

DATE _____ / _____ / _____

What is your favorite memory from when you were younger?

_____

_____

_____

Day 80

DATE _____ / _____ / _____

If you were a fairy, what kind of home would you live in? Describe it.

_____

_____

_____

Day 81

DATE _____ / _____ / _____

What did you do for your last birthday?

_____

_____

_____

Day 82

If you could invite anyone, real or imaginary, to a party, which three people would you invite? Why?

_____

_____

_____

Day 83

If you could beat a world record in something, what would you want it to be in? Why?

_____

_____

_____

Day 84

Would you rather be able to run as fast as a cheetah or swim as well as a dolphin? Why?

_____

_____

_____

Day 85

DATE _____ / _____ / _____

If you could share a piece of candy with every child in the world, what kind of candy would you share? Why?

_____

_____

_____

Day 86

DATE _____ / _____ / _____

If you met a magic genie, what are three things you would wish for? Why?

_____

_____

_____

Day 87

DATE _____ / _____ / _____

Have you ever lost something important? What was it?

_____

_____

_____

Day 88

What is something you would do if you were a superhero?

_____

_____

_____

Day 89

What is something you think is different now than when grown-ups were kids?

_____

_____

_____

Day 90

What is something you would like to learn more about? Why is it interesting to you?

_____

_____

_____

> "I can think whatever I like to think, I can play whatever I like to play, I can laugh whatever I like to laugh, there's nobody here but me."

—A. A. MILNE, *NOW WE ARE SIX*

Keep on writing. You are making some wonderful memories right now.

Day 91

DATE _____ / _____ / _____

How do you think the world would be different if children were tall and adults were short?

_____

_____

_____

Day 92

DATE _____ / _____ / _____

If you had a magic wand, what would you do with it?

_____

_____

_____

Day 93

DATE _____ / _____ / _____

Would you rather be able to understand everything animals say or have animals understand everything you say? Why?

_____

_____

_____

Day 94

DATE _____ / _____ / _____

What is something kids get to do that you would still like to do when you are grown up?

_____

_____

_____

Day 95

DATE _____ / _____ / _____

If you had a magic pencil that could make drawings come to life, what would you draw? Why?

_____

_____

_____

Day 96

DATE _____ / _____ / _____

Which movie or book world would you like to live in? Why?

_____

_____

_____

Day 97

If you were a dragon, what treasures would you collect? Why would you choose those things?

_____

_____

_____

Day 98

If you could invent a new flavor of ice cream, what would it be? Why?

_____

_____

_____

Day 99

If you could go back in time and meet your younger self, what would you say?

_____

_____

_____

Day 100

DATE _____ / _____ / _____

If you could invent a new kind of toy, what would it be like?

_____

_____

_____

Day 101

DATE _____ / _____ / _____

Is there someone you enjoy spending time with? What do you like about being with them?

_____

_____

_____

Day 102

DATE _____ / _____ / _____

If you could turn invisible, where would you go and what would you do?

_____

_____

_____

Day 103

DATE _____ / _____ / _____

If you were a bird, where would you build your nest? Why?

_____

_____

_____

Day 104

DATE _____ / _____ / _____

If you could go anywhere for one day, where would you go? Why?

_____

_____

_____

Day 105

DATE _____ / _____ / _____

What is something kind someone has done for you?

_____

_____

_____

Day 106

What imaginary creature would you like to have for a pet? Why?

_____

_____

_____

Day 107

What is something you would like to do when you are grown up? Why?

_____

_____

_____

Day 108

What is something you have done that you are proud of? Why are you proud of it?

_____

_____

_____

Day 109

DATE _____ / _____ / _____

If you had a pet parrot that could learn only one sentence, what would you teach it to say? Why?

_____

_____

_____

Day 110

DATE _____ / _____ / _____

Would you rather take care of a puppy or a baby? Why?

_____

_____

_____

Day 111

DATE _____ / _____ / _____

Think of a book you read recently that you really liked. What did you like about it?

_____

_____

_____

Day 112

If you could trade lives with someone for a day, who would it be and what would you do?

_____

_____

_____

Day 113

If you met a friendly monster, what would you do together?

_____

_____

_____

Day 114

What is something kind you have done for someone?

_____

_____

_____

Day 115

If you had one magical piece of clothing, what would it be and what would it do?

_____

_____

_____

Day 116

What is something you like about your friends?

_____

_____

_____

Day 117

If you wrote a book, what would you name the main character? Why would you choose that name?

_____

_____

_____

Day 118

DATE _____ / _____ / _____

If you could fly on a friendly dragon, where would you go?

_____

_____

_____

Day 119

DATE _____ / _____ / _____

If you had glasses that could see through walls, how would you use them?

_____

_____

_____

Day 120

DATE _____ / _____ / _____

What is something that makes you laugh?

_____

_____

_____

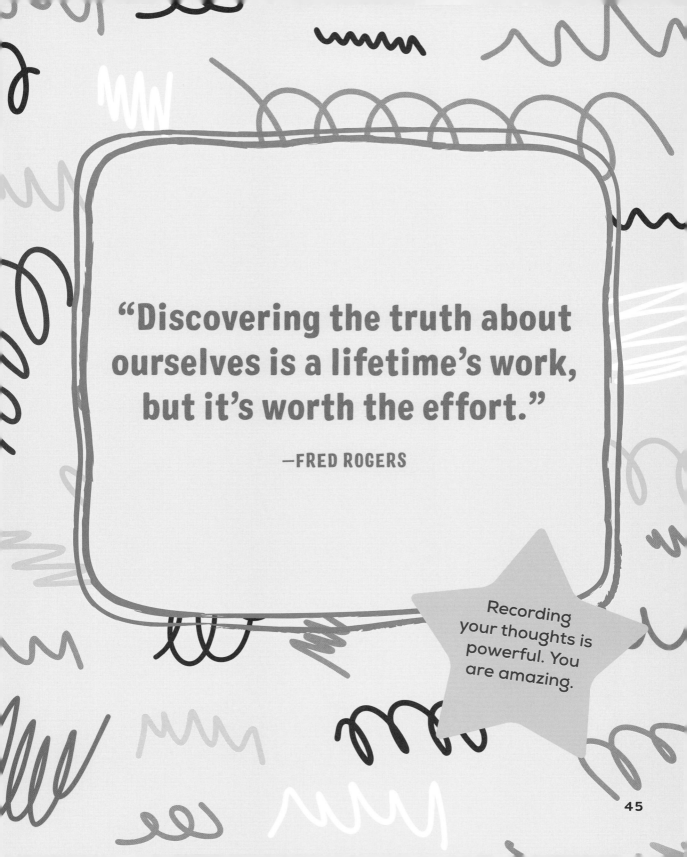

"Discovering the truth about ourselves is a lifetime's work, but it's worth the effort."

—FRED ROGERS

Recording your thoughts is powerful. You are amazing.

Day 121

DATE _____ / _____ / _____

If you were a sea creature, what kind of creature would you be? Why?

_____

_____

_____

Day 122

DATE _____ / _____ / _____

If you could paint a picture as big as a house, what would you paint?

_____

_____

_____

Day 123

DATE _____ / _____ / _____

What do you like best about yourself?

_____

_____

_____

Day 124

If you could change one thing about the world, what would it be?

_____

_____

_____

Day 125

Would you rather live in a world that is always daytime or a world that is always nighttime? Why?

_____

_____

_____

Day 126

What is something that is fun to share?

_____

_____

_____

Day 127

What do you think you would see if you were an astronaut in space?

_____

_____

_____

Day 128

Have you ever tried a food that you thought you wouldn't like but did?
What was it and what did you like about it?

_____

_____

_____

Day 129

Is there a quiet activity you like doing? What do you like about it?

_____

_____

_____

Day 130

DATE _____ / _____ / _____

What do you like to do when you have lots of energy?

_____

_____

_____

Day 131

DATE _____ / _____ / _____

How many people do you live with? What do you like about living with them?

_____

_____

_____

Day 132

DATE _____ / _____ / _____

What is a song you have stuck in your head right now? What do you like about it?

_____

_____

_____

Day 133

What is something that happened that surprised you?

_____

_____

_____

Day 134

If you were a photographer, what would you take pictures of?

_____

_____

_____

Day 135

What do you think you are very good at?

_____

_____

_____

Day 136

What is unique about you?

_____

_____

_____

Day 137

What do you like about the country you live in?

_____

_____

_____

Day 138

If you were a scientist, what would you want to study?

_____

_____

_____

Day 139

If you could eat only red foods or only green foods for the rest of your life, which would you pick? Why?

_____

_____

_____

Day 140

Would you rather take a ride on a motorcycle or in a hot-air balloon? Why?

_____

_____

_____

Day 141

If you could choose just three things to take with you to a deserted island, what would they be?

_____

_____

_____

Day 142

Would you rather ride a camel or a pony? Why?

_____

_____

_____

Day 143

If you could have a pet that was part one animal and part another (for example, half dog and half cat), which two animals would you combine? Why?

_____

_____

_____

Day 144

Would you rather have the power to never feel cold or to never feel hot? Why?

_____

_____

_____

Day 145

DATE _____ / _____ / _____

What is your favorite color in the rainbow? Why do you like it?

_____

_____

_____

Day 146

DATE _____ / _____ / _____

If you had a pet, what would you name it? Why?

_____

_____

_____

Day 147

DATE _____ / _____ / _____

If you could have a magical power for just one day, what power would you want?

_____

_____

_____

Day 148

If you were a bird, would you rather be a duck or an eagle? Why?

_____

_____

_____

Day 149

If you were a dog, would you rather be a big dog like a Great Dane or a little dog like a Chihuahua? Why?

_____

_____

_____

Day 150

Would you rather be a cave explorer or a circus performer? Why?

_____

_____

_____

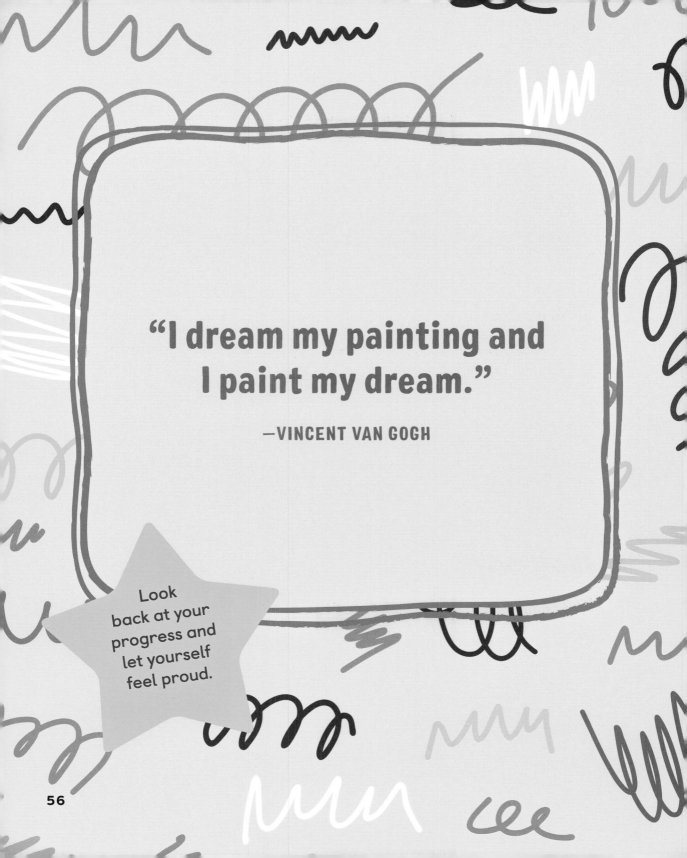

"I dream my painting and I paint my dream."

—VINCENT VAN GOGH

Look back at your progress and let yourself feel proud.

Day 151

DATE _____ / _____ / _____

If you met an alien who was trying to learn about our world, what are three things you would want to tell them about?

_____

_____

_____

Day 152

DATE _____ / _____ / _____

If a time traveler from 200 years ago came to your home, what do you think would be most surprising to them?

_____

_____

_____

Day 153

DATE _____ / _____ / _____

Some trees can live to be thousands of years old. What do you think it would be like if people lived that long?

_____

_____

_____

Day 154

DATE _____ / _____ / _____

Imagine you lived when your grandparents were young. What things might be different about your life?

_____

_____

_____

Day 155

DATE _____ / _____ / _____

Would you rather climb a mountain or swim across an enormous lake? Why?

_____

_____

_____

Day 156

DATE _____ / _____ / _____

Imagine you are the ruler of a magical kingdom. What is the first law you would make?

_____

_____

_____

Day 157

DATE _____ / _____ / _____

If you could design a playground, what kinds of things would it have?

_____

_____

_____

Day 158

DATE _____ / _____ / _____

If you were a bug, what kind would you want to be? Why?

_____

_____

_____

Day 159

DATE _____ / _____ / _____

What is something that makes you happy to think about? Why?

_____

_____

_____

Day 160

DATE _____ / _____ / _____

If you could turn the sky a different color, what color would you make it? Why?

_____

_____

_____

Day 161

DATE _____ / _____ / _____

If any kind of food could grow on trees, what kind of food tree would you want to plant? Why?

_____

_____

_____

Day 162

DATE _____ / _____ / _____

What is something nice you would like to do secretly for someone else?

_____

_____

_____

Day 163

What is something important that you have learned from a grown-up?

_____

_____

_____

Day 164

DATE _____ / _____ / _____

What is something interesting you learned about recently? Why did you find it interesting?

_____

_____

_____

Day 165

DATE _____ / _____ / _____

If you could have a dragon as a pet, what kinds of things do you think it might do?

_____

_____

_____

Day 166

If you could have one fantasy character to hang out with whenever you wanted, who would you choose?

_____

_____

_____

Day 167

If you could relive one day of your life so far, what day would you choose? Why?

_____

_____

_____

Day 168

If you had a musical instrument that was magical, what kind of instrument would it be and what would it do?

_____

_____

_____

Day 169

How would life be different if people swapped weekends—if they worked only on Saturday and Sunday and had fun for the rest of the week?

_____

_____

_____

Day 170

What is something that makes you feel less afraid when you are scared?

_____

_____

_____

Day 171

Would you rather live in a house built out of marshmallows or chocolate bars? Why?

_____

_____

_____

Day 172

If you could write a letter to any character in a book or a movie, who would you choose? What would you tell them?

_____

_____

_____

Day 173

If you could learn how to make any food, what would it be? Why?

_____

_____

_____

Day 174

If you could turn into an animal for just one day, what kind of animal would you be? Why?

_____

_____

_____

Day 175

DATE _____ / _____ / _____

Are you excited to grow up, or do you want to stay a kid? Why?

_____

_____

_____

Day 176

DATE _____ / _____ / _____

What is a game you like to play in a group? What do you like to play alone?

_____

_____

_____

Day 177

DATE _____ / _____ / _____

If you had one day where everyone did what you wanted, what would you do?

_____

_____

_____

Day 178

What is your favorite imaginary creature? What do you like about it?

_____

_____

_____

Day 179

How many people did you talk to today? What is something you talked about?

_____

_____

_____

Day 180

Would you rather live on a train or on a cruise ship? Why?

_____

_____

_____

> ## "Learning is beautiful."
>
> —NATALIE PORTMAN

Fantastic ideas here! Never stop writing.

Day 181

DATE _____ / _____ / _____

Can you imagine having four arms? How would that change the way you do things?

_____

_____

_____

Day 182

DATE _____ / _____ / _____

Where is your favorite place to be? Does it depend on what you're doing?

_____

_____

_____

Day 183

DATE _____ / _____ / _____

When is your favorite time of day (or night)? Why?

_____

_____

_____

Day 184

If you went to climb a mountain, who would you choose to go with you?

_____

_____

_____

Day 185

What do you like to do when you want some quiet time?

_____

_____

_____

Day 186

If you could build a robot to do one job for you, what task would you have it do?

_____

_____

_____

Day 187

DATE _____ / _____ / _____

If you could change your size for one day, would you rather be as tall as a giant or as small as a mouse?

_____

_____

_____

Day 188

DATE _____ / _____ / _____

If you were a made-up creature, would you be powerful and fierce or wise and gentle?

_____

_____

_____

Day 189

DATE _____ / _____ / _____

Imagine an animal called a **kwumpkin**. What kind of animal do you think it would be?

_____

_____

_____

Day 190

DATE _____ / _____ / _____

What is something that you like to do with other people? Why?

_____

_____

_____

Day 191

DATE _____ / _____ / _____

What is something that you like to do on your own?

_____

_____

_____

Day 192

DATE _____ / _____ / _____

What is something silly you have said or done?

_____

_____

_____

Day 193

What kind of music do you like? Do you like to sing or dance along to it?

_____

_____

_____

Day 194

Is there a place you haven't been to in a long time that you would like to go back to? Why do you want to go back?

_____

_____

_____

Day 195

Is there a place you have never been where you would like to go? Why do you want to go there?

_____

_____

_____

Day 196

DATE _____ / _____ / _____

What do you think you will be like when you are five years older than you are now?

_____

_____

_____

Day 197

DATE _____ / _____ / _____

If you could choose one of your toys to come to life, which one would you pick? Why would you choose that one?

_____

_____

_____

Day 198

DATE _____ / _____ / _____

Would you rather have a puppy or a kitten for a pet? Why?

_____

_____

Day 199

DATE _____ / _____ / _____

If you close your eyes and listen, what sounds can you hear right now?

_____

_____

_____

Day 200

DATE _____ / _____ / _____

What things do you remember from when you were really little?

_____

_____

_____

Day 201

DATE _____ / _____ / _____

How do you think things might be different if people were covered with fur?

_____

_____

_____

Day 202

DATE _____ / _____ / _____

How would you spend your time if you could do whatever you wanted for a week? Why?

_____

_____

_____

Day 203

DATE _____ / _____ / _____

If you met an alien, what would you ask them about their home planet?

_____

_____

_____

Day 204

DATE _____ / _____ / _____

What do you think it would be like to be a famous person? Who would you want to meet?

_____

_____

_____

Day 205

DATE _____ / _____ / _____

What is the most wonderful place you've ever been to? What did you love about this place?

_____

_____

_____

Day 206

DATE _____ / _____ / _____

What is your favorite dessert? Why?

_____

_____

_____

Day 207

DATE _____ / _____ / _____

Where is the farthest place from home you have ever been? What was it like?

_____

_____

_____

Day 208

DATE _____ / _____ / _____

If you could travel back to the time of the dinosaurs, what would you want to see?

_____

_____

_____

Day 209

DATE _____ / _____ / _____

Imagine you are living 100 years in the future. What is your life like?

_____

_____

_____

Day 210

DATE _____ / _____ / _____

If you could wish for one type of mythical creature to be real, which would you wish for? Why?

_____

_____

_____

"One child, one teacher, one book, and one pen can change the world."

—MALALA YOUSAFZAI

Way to go, writing in your journal! Using your own words is a great way to record things you do and think.

Day 211

DATE _____ / _____ / _____

What do you think a perfect friend would be like?

_____

_____

_____

Day 212

DATE _____ / _____ / _____

What is something creative that you like to do?

_____

_____

_____

Day 213

DATE _____ / _____ / _____

How would you describe the perfect pair of shoes for you?

_____

_____

_____

Day 214

DATE _____ / _____ / _____

What do you see when you look out the nearest window?

_____

_____

_____

Day 215

DATE _____ / _____ / _____

If someone from the future came back through a time machine to talk to you, what questions would you ask them?

_____

_____

_____

Day 216

DATE _____ / _____ / _____

If you could create a magic potion, what would it do?

_____

_____

_____

Day 217

DATE _____ / _____ / _____

If you could design a secret hideout, what would it be like?

_____

_____

_____

Day 218

DATE _____ / _____ / _____

If you made up a secret language, what would some of the words be?

_____

_____

_____

Day 219

DATE _____ / _____ / _____

Would you rather have a magic ring that could turn you invisible or one that could give you super speed? Why?

_____

_____

_____

Day 220

What do you know how to do that you can teach to other people? How did you learn to do that thing? What do you enjoy about it?

_____

_____

_____

Day 221

What do you think the world will be like when you are 80 years old?

_____

_____

_____

Day 222

Some animals can walk the day they are born. What do you think human babies would do if they could walk when they were born?

_____

_____

_____

Day 223

DATE _____ / _____ / _____

What is a kind of food you have never tried that you would like to try?

_____

_____

_____

Day 224

DATE _____ / _____ / _____

If you had a crystal ball that could show you anything happening right now, what would you look at?

_____

_____

_____

Day 225

DATE _____ / _____ / _____

If you could discover a planet, what color would it be? Who or what would live there?

_____

_____

_____

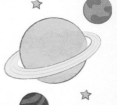

Day 226

DATE _____ / _____ / _____

If you could spend the whole day with just one person, who would it be? What would you do together?

_____

_____

_____

Day 227

DATE _____ / _____ / _____

What was the best thing you ate this week? Why did you like it?

_____

_____

_____

Day 228

DATE _____ / _____ / _____

What is a smell that you really like? Why do you like it?

_____

_____

_____

Day 229

DATE _____ / _____ / _____

Who is someone who helps you calm down when you're sad or angry? What do they do?

_____

_____

_____

Day 230

DATE _____ / _____ / _____

What is something hard that you really want to do? Why do you want to do it?

_____

_____

_____

Day 231

DATE _____ / _____ / _____

What is your favorite vegetable? Why do you like it?

_____

_____

_____

Day 232

DATE _____ / _____ / _____

What's one of your funniest dreams?

_____

_____

_____

Day 233

DATE _____ / _____ / _____

If you could choose what to dream about, what would you choose?

_____

_____

_____

Day 234

DATE _____ / _____ / _____

If you met the ruler of an ancient civilization, what is one question you would like to ask them?

_____

_____

_____

Day 235

Which two places would you live if you could spend half of the year in one place and the other half in another place? Why?

_____

_____

_____

Day 236

Imagine you could ride on the head of a dinosaur like a Brachiosaurus. What do you think your neighborhood would look like from way up there?

_____

_____

_____

Day 237

What is something you like to talk with your friends or family about? Why do you like talking about it?

_____

_____

_____

Day 238

DATE _____ / _____ / _____

Imagine you are writing a book where something surprising happens to your main character. What would that thing be? Why?

_____

_____

_____

Day 239

DATE _____ / _____ / _____

What is something you like to do that isn't on a screen? Why do you like that activity?

_____

_____

_____

Day 240

DATE _____ / _____ / _____

Would you rather spend a day on a beach or in a forest? Why?

_____

_____

_____

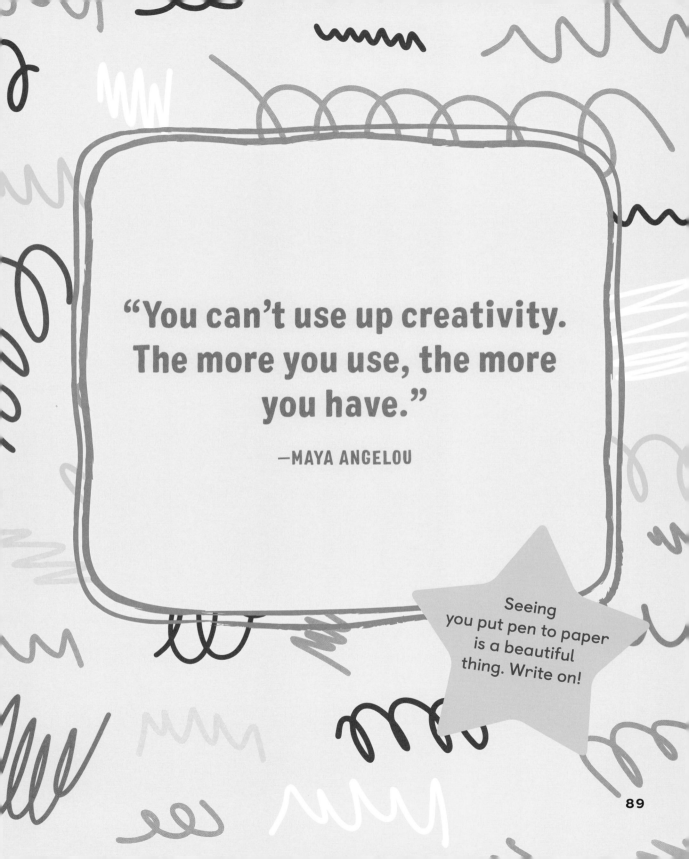

"You can't use up creativity. The more you use, the more you have."

—MAYA ANGELOU

Seeing you put pen to paper is a beautiful thing. Write on!

Day 241

DATE _____ / _____ / _____

What would life be like if gravity disappeared and people could float in the air?

_____

_____

_____

Day 242

DATE _____ / _____ / _____

What is something you saw or heard recently that you felt curious about?

_____

_____

_____

Day 243

DATE _____ / _____ / _____

What do you think stars look like up close? Do you have a favorite star or planet?

_____

_____

_____

Day 244

Would you like to be a pet, like a dog or a cat? Why or why not?

_____

_____

_____

Day 245

If your life were a cartoon, what do you think your character would be like?

_____

_____

_____

Day 246

If you lived in a castle, how would you use all the different rooms?

_____

_____

_____

Day 247

DATE _____ / _____ / _____

What is something that your family likes about you?

_____

_____

_____

Day 248

DATE _____ / _____ / _____

What is something you like about your family?

_____

_____

_____

Day 249

DATE _____ / _____ / _____

If you could add a class to your school day, what would you choose? Why?

_____

_____

_____

Day 250

DATE _____ / _____ / _____

If all the roads were turned into rivers, how would you like to get around?

_____

_____

_____

Day 251

DATE _____ / _____ / _____

What do you imagine animals think about the humans who live around them?

_____

_____

_____

Day 252

DATE _____ / _____ / _____

Can you describe a dream you remember having this week?

_____

_____

_____

Day 253

DATE _____ / _____ / _____

What is one way you like to calm yourself down when you feel frustrated?

_____

_____

_____

Day 254

DATE _____ / _____ / _____

If you could paint your fingernails any color, what color would you choose? Why?

_____

_____

_____

Day 255

DATE _____ / _____ / _____

Would you rather live in a city in the clouds or a city in the middle of the ocean? Why?

_____

_____

_____

Day 256

Would you rather be really good at climbing or really good at swimming? Why?

_____

_____

_____

Day 257

If you could know the answer to one question, what would you ask? Why?

_____

_____

_____

Day 258

If you were a plant, what kind of plant would you like to be? Why?

_____

_____

_____

Day 259

DATE _____ / _____ / _____

Would you rather have really good hearing or an excellent sense of smell? Why?

_____

_____

_____

Day 260

DATE _____ / _____ / _____

What's something you haven't done in a long time that you would like to do again? Why do you want to do it again?

_____

_____

_____

Day 261

DATE _____ / _____ / _____

What is your favorite thing to do with your family? Why did you choose that activity?

_____

_____

_____

Day 262

If you had wings, would they be feathery or scaly? Would they be furry or smooth? Why?

_____

_____

_____

Day 263

What would change about everyday life if humans didn't have eyes?

_____

_____

_____

Day 264

Write your own question for this journal. Now answer it!

_____

_____

_____

Day 265

DATE _____ / _____ / _____

What do you think it would be like to sleep for several months straight like a hibernating animal?

_____

_____

_____

Day 266

DATE _____ / _____ / _____

If you created a holiday, what would it be for? What would you name it and how would you celebrate?

_____

_____

_____

Day 267

DATE _____ / _____ / _____

If you named a country after yourself, what would it be called? Why?

_____

_____

_____

Day 268

DATE _____ / _____ / _____

What do you think it would be like to live in an upside-down house?

_____

_____

_____

Day 269

DATE _____ / _____ / _____

If you were in charge of building a school, what would it look like?

_____

_____

_____

Day 270

DATE _____ / _____ / _____

What are some ways your life might be different if you lived in a tree house?

_____

_____

_____

"It always seems impossible until it's done."

—NELSON MANDELA

Writing is an exploration of who you are! What will you learn about yourself next?

Day 271

DATE _____ / _____ / _____

If you had a cardboard box as big as a car, what would you do with it?

_____

_____

_____

Day 272

DATE _____ / _____ / _____

What colors would you paint your home if you got to choose all of the paint? Why would you choose those colors?

_____

_____

_____

Day 273

DATE _____ / _____ / _____

What would it be like if humans all had spikes like porcupines?

_____

_____

_____

Day 274

If you were a fairy, where would you sleep at night?

_____

_____

_____

Day 275

What do you think your life would be like if there were no grown-ups?

_____

_____

_____

Day 276

What is one way a friend or family member is different from you that makes them fun to spend time with?

_____

_____

_____

Day 277

DATE _____ / _____ / _____

What is something someone does for you all the time that you are grateful for?

_____

_____

_____

Day 278

DATE _____ / _____ / _____

What do you like to pretend to be when you play? Why?

_____

_____

_____

Day 279

DATE _____ / _____ / _____

If you found out you were secretly royalty, how do you think your life might change?

_____

_____

_____

Day 280

DATE _____ / _____ / _____

If you were the teacher, what would a school day look like?

_____

_____

_____

Day 281

DATE _____ / _____ / _____

What are three words you would like other people to think of when they think of you? Why?

_____

_____

_____

Day 282

DATE _____ / _____ / _____

Which family member do you think you are the most like? Why?

_____

_____

_____

Day 283

DATE _____ / _____ / _____

What is something you would like to surprise a friend or family member with? Why?

_____

_____

_____

Day 284

DATE _____ / _____ / _____

What is your favorite thing to eat for a snack? Why?

_____

_____

_____

Day 285

DATE _____ / _____ / _____

What was the best part of today?

_____

_____

_____

Day 286

If you had a flying horse, what would you name it? Why would you choose that name?

_____

_____

_____

Day 287

What would it be like if you had eyes in the back of your head?

_____

_____

_____

Day 288

What is something creative you could make out of only cardboard and tape?

_____

_____

_____

Day 289

If you discovered a new type of dinosaur, what would you name it? Why would you choose that name?

_____

_____

_____

Day 290

DATE _____ / _____ / _____

What is something you like to do when you get ready for bed?

_____

_____

_____

Day 291

DATE _____ / _____ / _____

If you could invent a new kind of pizza, what would you put on it? Why?

_____

_____

_____

Day 292

DATE _____ / _____ / _____

If you could choose two people to spend a year with on a space station, who would you choose? Why?

_____

_____

_____

Day 293

DATE _____ / _____ / _____

Would you rather have a pet big enough for you to ride on or small enough to fit in your pocket?

_____

_____

_____

Day 294

DATE _____ / _____ / _____

Would you rather eat only fruits or only vegetables? Why?

_____

_____

_____

Day 295

Can you imagine an unusual outfit that would be fun to wear? What would it be like?

_____

_____

_____

Day 296

If you could drive a car, what kind of car would you want to drive? Why?

_____

_____

_____

Day 297

What is something you think it would be fun to set a world record in? Why?

_____

_____

_____

Day 298

DATE _____ / _____ / _____

If someone gave you a million dollars, what would you do with it?

_____

_____

_____

Day 299

DATE _____ / _____ / _____

If you could live in any year in history, what year would it be and why?

_____

_____

_____

Day 300

DATE _____ / _____ / _____

If you could make a law, what would it say?

_____

_____

_____

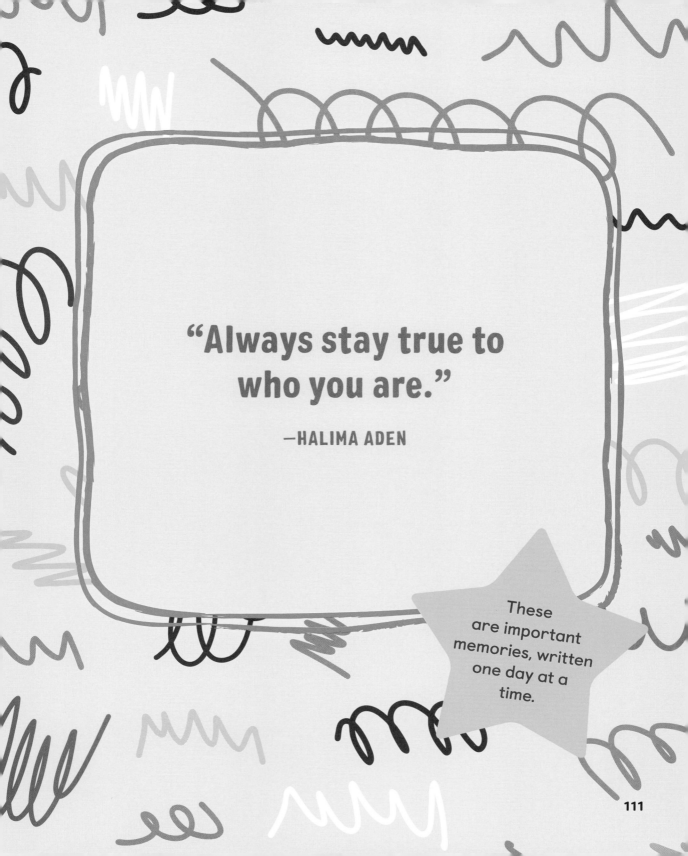

"Always stay true to who you are."

—HALIMA ADEN

These are important memories, written one day at a time.

Day 301

DATE _____ / _____ / _____

Pretend you are a mouse exploring your room. What would you see and do?

_____

_____

_____

Day 302

DATE _____ / _____ / _____

What is one goal you have for this year? What are some things you can do to work toward that goal?

_____

_____

_____

Day 303

DATE _____ / _____ / _____

What is the hardest thing you've ever done in your life?

_____

_____

_____

Day 304

Can you imagine what a gathering of fairies might eat for a feast? Describe their food.

_____

_____

_____

Day 305

Would you rather be a superhero or a supervillain? Why?

_____

_____

_____

Day 306

If you could be famous, what would you like to be famous for?

_____

_____

_____

Day 307

DATE _____ / _____ / _____

What is your favorite season? Why do you like that season?

_____

_____

_____

Day 308

DATE _____ / _____ / _____

What do you like best about growing up?

_____

_____

_____

Day 309

DATE _____ / _____ / _____

If you could invent a new sport, what would it be called and how would people play it?

_____

_____

_____

Day 310

What is something you have done that made someone else happy?

_____

_____

_____

Day 311

DATE _____ / _____ / _____

Imagine a distant planet where the aliens have pets called **zoglebips**. What do you think a zoglebip would be like?

_____

_____

_____

Day 312

DATE _____ / _____ / _____

What was something you did today? Try to make it sound really exciting (even if it wasn't)!

_____

_____

_____

Day 313

If you could say only one word out loud for the rest of your life, what would it be? Why would you choose that word?

_____

_____

_____

Day 314

How do you think things might be different if people never grew hair on top of their heads?

_____

_____

_____

Day 315

What does your favorite pair of pajamas look like? Why are they your favorite?

_____

_____

_____

Day 316

If you and your family and friends were all cats, what would you spend your days doing?

_____

_____

_____

Day 317

If you had your own private helicopter, how would you use it?

_____

_____

_____

Day 318

What would you do if you could see in the dark?

_____

_____

_____

Day 319

DATE _____ / _____ / _____

What are some differences between the sounds you hear at night and the sounds you hear during the daytime where you live?

_____

_____

_____

Day 320

DATE _____ / _____ / _____

If you had to eat the same thing for every meal for one week, what food would you choose? Why?

_____

_____

_____

Day 321

DATE _____ / _____ / _____

What are the first things you usually do after you get up in the morning?

_____

_____

_____

Day 322

DATE _____ / _____ / _____

If you could be an animal keeper at the zoo, which animals would you like to take care of? Why would you choose those animals?

_____

_____

_____

Day 323

DATE _____ / _____ / _____

If you were a schoolteacher, what field trip would you like to take your class on? Why would you choose that trip?

_____

_____

_____

Day 324

DATE _____ / _____ / _____

Can you share a joke that you found funny? Or make up your own!

_____

_____

_____

Day 325

DATE _____ / _____ / _____

If you were an architect, what kind of building would you most like to design? Why?

_____

_____

_____

Day 326

DATE _____ / _____ / _____

If you could breathe underwater, what would you like to explore in the ocean? Why?

_____

_____

_____

Day 327

DATE _____ / _____ / _____

If you close your eyes, what is the quietest sound you can hear? Where is it coming from?

_____

_____

_____

Day 328

DATE _____ / _____ / _____

If you had the power to make yourself invisible, how might you secretly help someone?

_____

_____

_____

Day 329

DATE _____ / _____ / _____

If the moon were made of cheese, what kind of cheese do you think it would be made of? Why?

_____

_____

_____

Day 330

DATE _____ / _____ / _____

Would you rather eat only spicy food or only bland food? Why?

_____

_____

_____

"**Just try new things.
Don't be afraid.**"

—MICHELLE OBAMA

You have a lot
to say. That is
awesome!

Day 331

If you had $1,000 to spend at one store, which store would you go to and what would you buy? Why?

_____

_____

_____

Day 332

If you could hire an artist to paint a mural on your bedroom wall, what kind of picture would you want them to paint? Why?

_____

_____

_____

Day 333

If you were writing a letter to your future grandchildren, what would you tell them about the way things were when you were a child?

_____

_____

_____

Day 334

Describe some interesting plants or animals that you see when you walk outside and look around.

_____

_____

_____

Day 335

If you had a magic ring with a single gem, what color gem would it be? What would the ring do?

_____

_____

_____

Day 336

Talk about a time when you felt really happy. Why were you so happy?

_____

_____

_____

Day 337

DATE _____ / _____ / _____

If you could make something out of play dough and have it come to life, what would you make? Why?

_____

_____

_____

Day 338

DATE _____ / _____ / _____

If a kid from another country was coming to visit your area, what would you take them to see or do? Why?

_____

_____

_____

Day 339

DATE _____ / _____ / _____

What are three things you like about someone in your family?

_____

_____

_____

Day 340

If you were a reporter interviewing someone important, what questions would you ask them?

_____

_____

_____

Day 341

If you could spend one day doing whatever you wanted, what would you do?

_____

_____

_____

Day 342

What do you like to do to keep from being bored when you are waiting for something?

_____

_____

_____

Day 343

DATE _____ / _____ / _____

Is there anything you are looking forward to in the next month? What makes you excited about it?

_____

_____

_____

Day 344

DATE _____ / _____ / _____

If you were an explorer going into the jungle to find the ruins of a lost city, what would you take with you? Why?

_____

_____

_____

Day 345

DATE _____ / _____ / _____

What would you do if you woke up one morning and found a monkey climbing around your room?

_____

_____

_____

Day 346

Do you like surprises, or do you like to know what is going to happen before it happens? Why?

_____

_____

_____

Day 347

What is something you are grateful for?

_____

_____

_____

Day 348

If you had your own store, what kinds of things would you sell?

_____

_____

_____

Day 349

DATE _____ / _____ / _____

Can you describe the room you are in right now?

_____

_____

_____

Day 350

DATE _____ / _____ / _____

If you designed a video game, what would it be like?

_____

_____

_____

Day 351

DATE _____ / _____ / _____

What do you think is the most important thing to do every day? Why?

_____

_____

_____

Day 352

Talk about a time when you did something that was hard for you. Did you feel proud when you finished it?

_____

_____

_____

Day 353

If you could turn into one kind of animal whenever you wanted, what animal would you choose? Why?

_____

_____

_____

Day 354

Imagine a mystery creature that might live in your area. What kind of creature would it be?

_____

_____

_____

Day 355

DATE _____ / _____ / _____

If you built a museum, what would you exhibit in it?

_____

_____

_____

Day 356

DATE _____ / _____ / _____

If you were going far away and could only take one of your toys with you, which toy would you choose? Why?

_____

_____

_____

Day 357

DATE _____ / _____ / _____

Do you think you would rather be really organized or really creative? Why? Do you think you could be both?

_____

_____

_____

Day 358

DATE _____ / _____ / _____

If you could grow any kind of plant in your room, what would you grow? Why?

_____

_____

_____

Day 359

DATE _____ / _____ / _____

What is an activity you haven't tried before but would like to try? Why would you like to try it?

_____

_____

_____

Day 360

DATE _____ / _____ / _____

If you had the power to control fire, air, earth, or water, which element would you want to control? Why?

_____

_____

_____

Day 361

DATE _____ / _____ / _____

If you found a pot of gold, what would you do with it?

_____

_____

_____

Day 362

DATE _____ / _____ / _____

If you had the power to change one thing about the world to make it a better place, what would you change? Why?

_____

_____

_____

Day 363

DATE _____ / _____ / _____

What are your most comfortable clothes? What makes them so comfy?

_____

_____

_____

Day 364

Is there something about yourself that you think is unique? What is it, and how does it make you different from other people?

_____

_____

_____

Day 365

Would you rather be able to hear through walls or see in the dark? Why?

_____

_____

_____

Day 366

Describe someone you admire. Why do you admire them?

_____

Bonus
Question!

_____

"The future belongs to those who believe in the beauty of their dreams."

—ELEANOR ROOSEVELT

You've written about so many interesting things! Keep up the good work.

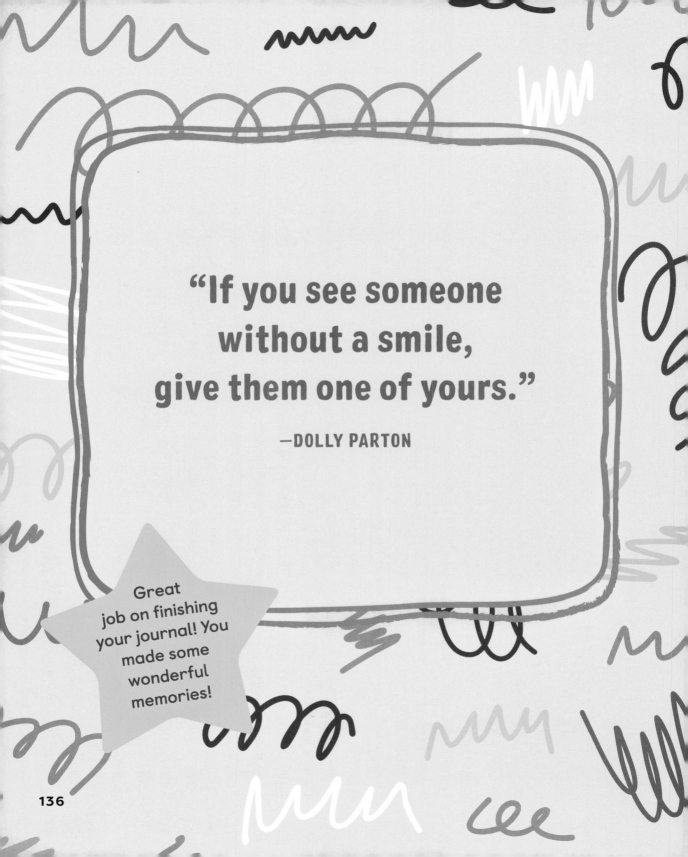

"If you see someone
without a smile,
give them one of yours."

—DOLLY PARTON

Great job on finishing your journal! You made some wonderful memories!

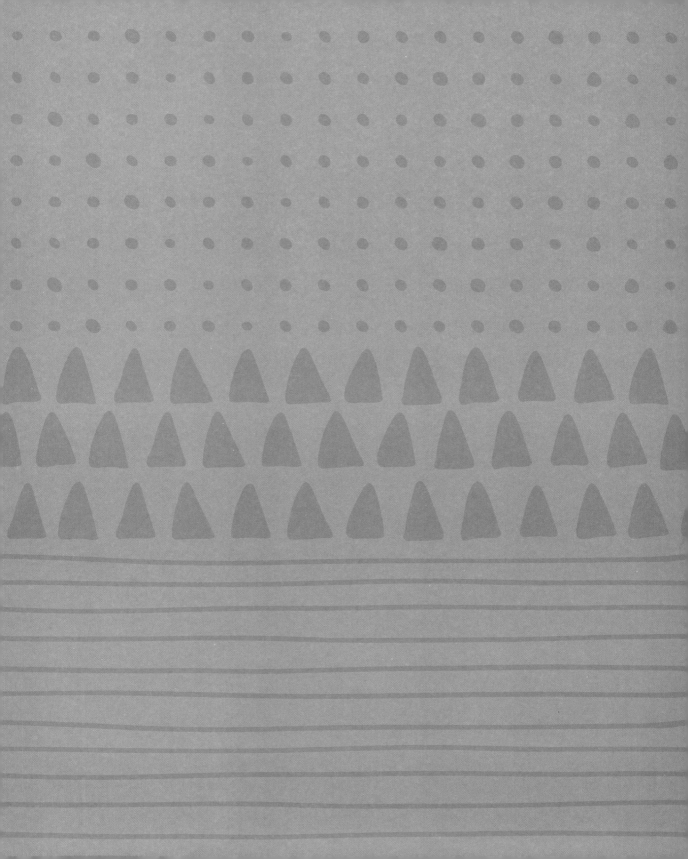

Acknowledgments

This book would not be possible without the incredible imaginations of Rachel, Nathanael, Eva, Samuel, Hannah, Josiah, Luke, Sarah, and Anna—all of whom helped me think up questions. Many thanks to the incredible publishing staff who worked to edit, illustrate, and bring this book to life.

About the Author

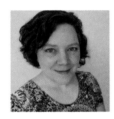 MaryAnne Kochenderfer enjoyed a wonderful childhood, first on a corn farm in Utah, and then living in Guatemala, France, Bolivia, and Austria. She chronicled those adventures in her own childhood journals, which she enjoys reading as an adult.

MaryAnne now lives in California with her husband, Mike, and their four amazing children. She loves traveling with her kids, and they go on a road trip most summers. She writes about crafts, activities, and family travel on her blog at MamaSmiles.com. MaryAnne spends her free time with her family and playing her guitar and singing. A childhood cancer survivor, MaryAnne believes in making memories every single day.